Affordable Plant Based Diet Plan

Change your Lifestyle with This Ultimate Cookbook

Joanna Vinson

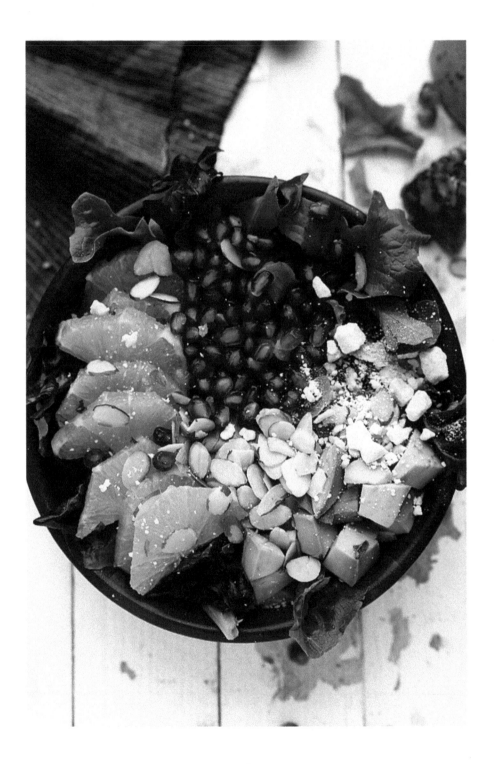

TABLE OF CONTENTS

Warm Pomegranate Punch

Preparation Time: 15-30 minutes | Cooking Time: 2 hours and 15 minutes | Servings: 10

Ingredients:

• 3 cinnamon sticks, each about 3 inches long

• 12 whole cloves

• 1/2 cup of coconut sugar

• 1/3 cup of lemon juice

• 32 fluid ounce of pomegranate juice

• 32 fluid ounce of apple juice, unsweetened

• 16 fluid ounce of brewed tea

Directions:

• Using a 4-quart slow cooker, pour the lemon juice, pomegranate, juice apple juice, tea, and then sugar.

• Wrap the whole cloves and cinnamon stick in a cheesecloth, tie its corners with a string, and immerse it in the liquid present in the slow cooker.

• Then cover it with the lid, plug in the slow cooker and let it cook at the low heat setting for 3 hours or until it is heated thoroughly.

• When done, discard the cheesecloth bag and serve it hot or cold.

Nutrition:

Calories:253 Cal | Carbohydrates:58g | Protein:7g | Fats:2g | Fiber:3g.

Rich Truffle Hot Chocolate

Preparation Time: 15-30 minutes | Cooking Time: 1 hour and 10 minutes | Servings: 4

Ingredients:

- 1/3 cup of cocoa powder, unsweetened

- 1/3 cup of coconut sugar

- 1/8 teaspoon of salt

- 1/8 teaspoon of ground cinnamon

- 1 teaspoon of vanilla extract, unsweetened

- 32 fluid ounce of coconut milk

Directions:

- Using a 2 quarts slow cooker, add all the ingredients, and stir properly.

- Cover it with the lid, then plug in the slow cooker and cook it for 2 hours on the high heat

setting or until it is heated thoroughly.

- When done, serve right away.

Nutrition:

Calories:67 Cal | Carbohydrates:13g | Protein:2g | Fats:2g |
Fiber:2. 3g.

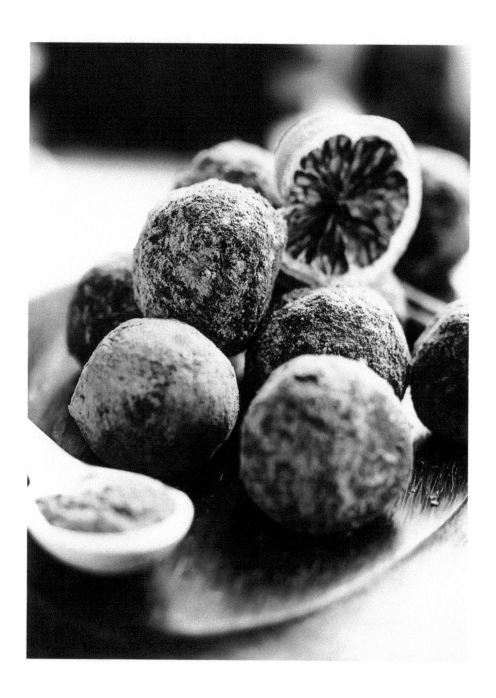

Warm Spiced Lemon Drink

Preparation Time: 15-30 minutes | Cooking Time: 2 hours and 10 minutes | Servings: 12

Ingredients:

- 1 cinnamon stick, about 3 inches long

- 1/2 teaspoon of whole cloves

- 2 cups of coconut sugar

- 4 fluid of ounce pineapple juice

- 1/2 cup and 2 tablespoons of lemon juice

- 12 fluid ounce of orange juice

- 2 1/2 quarts of water

Directions:

- Pour water into a 6-quarts slow cooker and stir the sugar and lemon juice properly.

- Wrap the cinnamon, the whole cloves in cheesecloth, and tie its corners with string.

• Immerse this cheesecloth bag in the liquid present in the slow cooker and cover it with the lid.

• Then plug in the slow cooker and let it cook on a high heat setting for 2 hours or until it is heated thoroughly.

• When done, discard the cheesecloth bag and serve the drink hot or cold.

Nutrition:

Calories:15 Cal | Carbohydrates:3. 2g | Protein:0. 1g | Fats:0g | Fiber:0g.

Ultimate Mulled Wine

Preparation Time: 15-30 minutes | Cooking Time: 35 minutes | Servings: 6

Ingredients:

- 1 cup of cranberries, fresh

- 2 oranges, juiced

- 1 tablespoon of whole cloves

- 2 cinnamon sticks, each about 3 inches long

- 1 tablespoon of star anise

- 1/3 cup of honey

- 8 fluid ounce of apple cider

- 8 fluid ounce of cranberry juice

- 24 fluid ounce of red wine

Directions:

- Using a 4 quarts slow cooker, add all the ingredients, and stir properly.

• Cover it with the lid, then plug in the slow cooker and cook it for 30 minutes on the high heat

setting or until it gets warm thoroughly.

• When done, strain the wine and serve right away.

Nutrition:

Calories:202 Cal | Carbohydrates:25g | Protein:0g | Fats:0g | Fiber:0g.

Pleasant Lemonade

Preparation Time: 15-30 minutes | Cooking Time: 3 hours and 15 minutes | Servings: 10 servings

Ingredients:

- Cinnamon sticks for serving

- 2 cups of coconut sugar

- 1/4 cup of honey

- 3 cups of lemon juice. fresh

- 32 fluid ounce of water

Directions:

- Using a 4-quarts slow cooker, place all the ingredients except for the cinnamon sticks and stir properly.

- Cover it with the lid, then plug in the slow cooker and cook it for 3 hours on the low heat setting or until it is heated thoroughly.

- When done, stir properly and serve with the cinnamon sticks.

Nutrition:

Calories:146 Cal | Carbohydrates:34g | Protein:0g | Fats:0g | Fiber:0g.

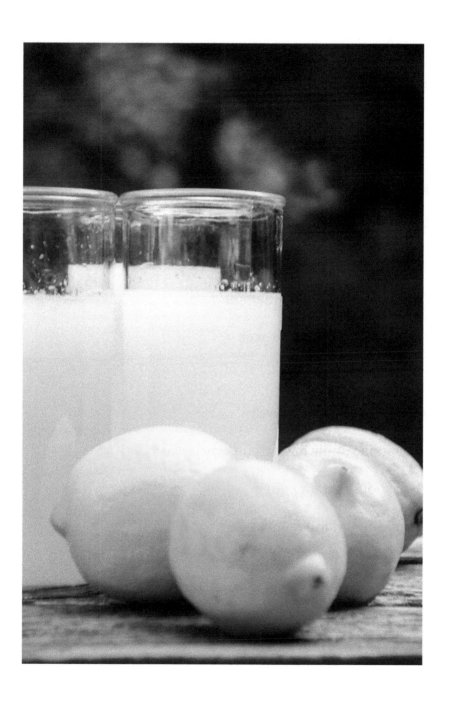

Pumpkin Spice Frappuccino

Preparation Time: 5 minutes | Cooking Time: 0 minute | Servings: 2

Ingredients:

• ½ teaspoon ground ginger

• 1/8 teaspoon allspice

• ½ teaspoon ground cinnamon

• 2 tablespoons coconut sugar

• 1/8 teaspoon nutmeg

• ¼ teaspoon ground cloves

• 1 teaspoon vanilla extract, unsweetened

• 2 teaspoons instant coffee

• 2 cups almond milk, unsweetened

• 1 cup of ice cubes

Directions:

• Place all the ingredients in the order in a food processor or blender and then pulse for 2 to 3 minutes at high speed until smooth.

• Pour the Frappuccino into two glasses and then serve.

Nutrition:

Calories: 490 | Fat: 9g | Protein: 12g | Sugar: 11g

Cookie Dough Milkshake

Preparation Time: 5 minutes | Cooking Time: 0 minute | Servings: 2

Ingredients:

• 2 tablespoons cookie dough

• 5 dates, pitted

• 2 teaspoons chocolate chips

• 1/2 teaspoon vanilla extract, unsweetened

• 1/2 cup almond milk, unsweetened

• 1 ½ cup almond milk ice cubes

Directions:

• Place all the ingredients in the order in a food processor or blender and then pulse for 2 to 3 minutes at high speed until smooth.

• Pour the milkshake into two glasses and then serve with some cookie dough balls.

Nutrition:

Calories: 240 | Fat: 13g | Protein: 21g | Sugar: 9g

Strawberry and Hemp Smoothie

Preparation Time: 5 minutes | Cooking Time: 0 minute | Servings: 2

Ingredients:

- 3 cups fresh strawberries

- 2 tablespoons hemp seeds

- 1/2 teaspoon vanilla extract, unsweetened

- 1/8 teaspoon sea salt

- 2 tablespoons maple syrup

- 1 cup vegan yogurt

- 1 cup almond milk, unsweetened

- 1 cup of ice cubes

- 2 tablespoons hemp protein

Directions:

- Place all the ingredients in the order in a food processor or blender, except for protein powder, and then pulse for 2 to 3 minutes at high speed until smooth.

• Pour the smoothie into two glasses and then serve.

Nutrition:

Calories: 510 | Fat: 18g | Protein: 26g | Sugar: 12g

Blueberry, Hazelnut, and Hemp Smoothie

Preparation Time: 5 minutes | Cooking Time: 0 minute | Servings: 2

Ingredients:

• 2 tablespoons hemp seeds

• 1 ½ cups frozen blueberries

• 2 tablespoons chocolate protein powder

• 1/2 teaspoon vanilla extract, unsweetened

• 2 tablespoons chocolate hazelnut butter

• 1 small frozen banana

• 3/4 cup almond milk

Directions:

• Place all the ingredients in the order in a food processor or blender and then pulse for 2 to 3 minutes at high speed until smooth.

• Pour the smoothie into two glasses and then serve.

Nutrition:

Calories: 195 | Fat: 14g | Protein: 36g | Sugar: 10g

Mango Lassi

Preparation Time: 5 minutes | Cooking Time: 0 minute | Servings: 2

Ingredients:

- 1 ¼ cup mango pulp

- 1 tablespoon coconut sugar

- 1/8 teaspoon salt

- 1/2 teaspoon lemon juice

- 1/4 cup almond milk, unsweetened

- 1/4 cup chilled water

- 1 cup cashew yogurt

Directions:

• Place all the ingredients in the order in a food processor or blender and then pulse for 2 to 3 minutes at high speed until smooth.

• Pour the lassi into two glasses and then serve.

Nutrition:

Calories: 420 | Fat: 12g | Protein: 23g | Sugar: 13g

Mocha Chocolate Shake

Preparation Time: 5 minutes | Cooking Time: 0 minute | Servings: 2

Ingredients:

- 1/4 cup hemp seeds

- 2 teaspoons cocoa powder, unsweetened

- 1/2 cup dates, pitted

- 1 tablespoon instant coffee powder

- 2 tablespoons flax seeds

- 2 1/2 cups almond milk, unsweetened

- 1/2 cup crushed ice

Directions:

- Place all the ingredients in the order in a food processor or blender and then pulse for 2 to 3 minutes at high speed until smooth.

- Pour the smoothie into two glasses and then serve.

Nutrition:

- Calories: 432 | Fat: 18g | Protein: 14g | Sugar: 12g

Chard, Lettuce, and Ginger Smoothie

Preparation Time: 5 minutes | Cooking Time: 0 minute | Servings: 2

Ingredients:

- 10 Chard leaves, chopped
- inch piece of ginger, chopped
- 10 lettuce leaves, chopped
- ½ teaspoon black salt
- 2 pear, chopped
- 2 teaspoons coconut sugar
- ¼ teaspoon ground black pepper
- ¼ teaspoon salt
- 2 tablespoons lemon juice
- 2 cups of water

Directions:

- Place all the ingredients in the order in a food processor or blender and then pulse for 2 to 3 minutes at high speed until smooth.

- Pour the smoothie into two glasses and then serve.

Nutrition:

Calories: 240 | Fat: 4g | Protein: 16g | Sugar: 3g

Red Beet, Pear, and Apple Smoothie

Preparation Time: 5 minutes | Cooking Time: 0 minute | Servings: 2

Ingredients:

- 1/2 of medium beet, peeled, chopped

- 1 tablespoon chopped cilantro

- 1 orange, juiced

- 1 medium pear, chopped

- 1 medium apple, cored, chopped

- 1/4 teaspoon ground black pepper

- 1/8 teaspoon rock salt

- 1 teaspoon coconut sugar

- 1/4 teaspoons salt

- 1 cup of water

Directions:

• Place all the ingredients in the order in a food processor or blender and then pulse for 2 to 3 minutes at high speed until smooth.

• Pour the smoothie into two glasses and then serve.

Nutrition:

Calories: 240 | Fat: 4g | Protein: 16g | Sugar: 3g

Berry and Yogurt Smoothie

Preparation Time: 5 minutes | Cooking Time: 0 minute | Servings: 2

Ingredients:

• 2 small bananas

• 3 cups frozen mixed berries

• 1 ½ cup cashew yogurt

• 1/2 teaspoon vanilla extract, unsweetened

• 1/2 cup almond milk, unsweetened

Directions:

• Place all the ingredients in the order in a food processor or blender and then pulse for 2 to 3 minutes at high speed until smooth.

• Pour the smoothie into two glasses and then serve.

Nutrition:

Calories: 291 | Fat: 9g | Protein: 17g | Sugar: 5g

Chocolate and Cherry Smoothie

Preparation Time: 5 minutes | Cooking Time: 0 minute | Servings: 2

Ingredients:

• 4 cups frozen cherries

• 2 tablespoons cocoa powder

• 1 scoop of protein powder

• 1 teaspoon maple syrup

• 2 cups almond milk, unsweetened

Directions:

• Place all the ingredients in the order in a food processor or blender and then pulse for 2 to 3 minutes at high speed until smooth.

• Pour the smoothie into two glasses and then serve.

Nutrition:

Calories: 247 | Fat: 3g | Protein: 18g | Sugar: 3g

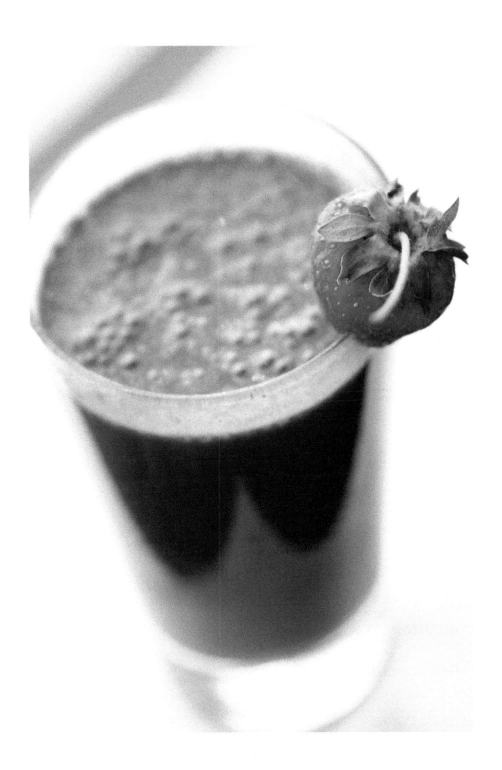

Banana Weight Loss Juice

Preparation Time: 10 minutes | Cooking Time: 0 minutes | Servings: 1

Ingredients:

• Water (1/3 C.)

• Apple (1, Sliced)

• Orange (1, Sliced)

• Banana (1, Sliced)

• Lemon Juice (1 T.)

Directions:

• Simply place everything into your blender, blend on high for twenty seconds, and then pour into your glass.

Nutrition:

Calories: 289 | Total Carbohydrate: 2 g | Cholesterol: 3 mg | Total Fat: 17 g | Fiber: 2 g | Protein: 7 g | Sodium: 163 mg

Vitamin Green Smoothie

Preparation Time: 5 minutes | Cooking Time: 5 minutes | Servings: 2

Ingredients:

- 1 cup milk or juice

- 1 cup spinach or kale

- ½ cup plain yogurt

- 1 kiwi

- 1 Tbsp chia or flax

- 1 tsp vanilla

Directions:

- Mix the milk or juice and greens until smooth. Add the remaining ingredients and continue blending until smooth again.

- Enjoy your delicious drink!

Nutrition:

Calories 397 | Fat 36.4 g | Carbohydrates 4 g | Sugar 1 g | Protein 14.7 g | Cholesterol 4 mg

Strawberry Grapefruit Smoothie

Preparation Time: 5 minutes | Cooking Time: 5 minutes | Servings: 2

Ingredients:

• 1 banana

• ½ cup strawberries, frozen

• 1 grapefruit

• ¼ cup milk

• ¼ cup plain yogurt

• 2 Tbsp honey

• ½ tsp ginger, chopped

Directions:

• Using a mixer, blend all the ingredients.

• When smooth, top your drink with a slice of grapefruit and enjoy it!

Nutrition:

Calories 233 | Fat 7.9 g | Carbohydrates 3.2 g | Sugar 0.1 g |
Protein 35.6 g | Cholesterol 32 mg

Spiced Buttermilk

Preparation Time: 5 minutes | Cooking Time: 0 minute | Servings: 2

Ingredients:

- 3/4 teaspoon ground cumin

- 1/4 teaspoon sea salt

- 1/8 teaspoon ground black pepper

- 2 mint leaves

- 1/8 teaspoon lemon juice

- ¼ cup cilantro leaves

- 1 cup of chilled water

- 1 cup vegan yogurt, unsweetened

- Ice as needed

Directions:

- Place all the ingredients in the order in a food processor or blender, except for cilantro and ¼ teaspoon cumin, and then pulse for 2 to 3 minutes at high speed until smooth.

• Pour the milk into glasses, top with cilantro and cumin, and then serve.

Nutrition:

Calories: 211 | Total Carbohydrate: 7 g | Cholesterol: 13 mg | Total Fat: 18 g | Fiber: 3 g | Protein: 17 g | Sodium: 289 mg

Turmeric Lassi

Preparation Time: 5 minutes | Cooking Time: 0 minute | Servings: 2

Ingredients:

- 1 teaspoon grated ginger

- 1/8 teaspoon ground black pepper

- 1 teaspoon turmeric powder

- 1/8 teaspoon cayenne

- 1 tablespoon coconut sugar

- 1/8 teaspoon salt

- 1 cup vegan yogurt

- 1 cup almond milk

Directions:

- Place all the ingredients in the order in a food processor or blender and then pulse for 2 to 3 minutes at high speed until smooth.

- Pour the lassi into two glasses and then serve.

Nutrition:

Calories: 392 | Fat: 10g | Protein: 18g | Sugar: 8g

Brownie Batter Orange Chia Shake

Preparation Time: 5 minutes | Cooking Time: 0 minute | Servings: 2

Ingredients:

- 2 tablespoons cocoa powder
- 3 tablespoons chia seeds
- ¼ teaspoon salt
- 4 tablespoons chocolate chips
- 4 teaspoons coconut sugar
- ½ teaspoon orange zest
- ½ teaspoon vanilla extract, unsweetened
- 2 cup almond milk

Directions:

- Place all the ingredients in the order in a food processor or blender and then pulse for 2 to 3 minutes at high speed until smooth.

• Pour the smoothie into two glasses and then serve.

Nutrition:

Calories: 290 | Fat: 11g | Protein: 20g | Sugar: 9g

Saffron Pistachio Beverage

Preparation Time: 5 minutes | Cooking Time: 0 minute | Servings: 2

Ingredients:

• 8 strands of saffron

• 1 tablespoon cashews

• 1/4 teaspoon ground ginger

• 2 tablespoons pistachio

• 1/8 teaspoon cloves

• 1/4 teaspoon ground black pepper

• 1/4 teaspoon cardamom powder

• 3 tablespoons coconut sugar

• 1/4 teaspoon cinnamon

• 1/8 teaspoon fennel seeds

• 1/4 teaspoon poppy seeds

Directions:

• Place all the ingredients in the order in a food processor or blender and then pulse for 2 to 3 minutes at high speed until smooth.

 • Pour the smoothie into two glasses and then serve.

Nutrition:

Calories: 394 | Fat: 5g | Protein: 12g | Sugar: 4g

Mexican Hot Chocolate Mix

Preparation Time: 5 minutes | Cooking Time: 0 minute | Servings: 2

Ingredients:

For the Hot Chocolate Mix:

• 1/3 cup chopped dark chocolate

• 1/8 teaspoon cayenne

• 1/8 teaspoon salt

• 1/2 teaspoon cinnamon

• 1/4 cup coconut sugar

• 1 teaspoon cornstarch

• 3 tablespoons cocoa powder

• 1/2 teaspoon vanilla extract, unsweetened

For Servings:

• 2 cups milk, warmed

Directions:

• Place all the ingredients of the hot chocolate mix in the order in a food processor or blender and then pulse for 2 to 3 minutes at high speed until ground.

• Stir 2 tablespoons of the chocolate mix into a glass of milk until combined and then serve.

Nutrition:

Calories: 160 | Fat: 6g | Protein: 26g | Sugar: 7g

Inspirational Orange Smoothie

Preparation Time: 5 minutes | Cooking Time: 5 minutes | Servings: 1

Ingredients:

- 4 mandarin oranges, peeled

- 1 banana, sliced and frozen

- ½ cup non-fat Greek yogurt

- ¼ cup of coconut water

- 1 tsp vanilla extract

- 5 ice cubes

Directions:

- Using a mixer, whisk all the ingredients.

- Enjoy your drink!

Nutrition:

Calories 256 | Fat 13.3 g | Carbohydrates 0 g | Sugar 0 g | Protein 34.5 g | Cholesterol 78 mg

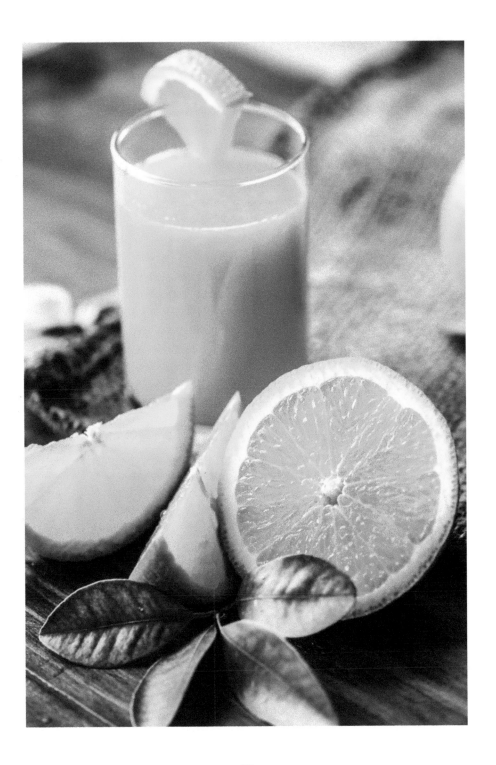

High Protein Blueberry Banana Smoothie

Preparation Time: 5 minutes | Cooking Time: 5 minutes | Servings: 2

Ingredients:

- 1 cup blueberries, frozen

- 2 ripe bananas

- 1 cup of water

- 1 tsp vanilla extract

- 2 Tbsp chia seeds

- ½ cup cottage cheese

- 1 tsp lemon zest

Directions:

- Put all the smoothie ingredients into the blender and whisk until smooth.

- Enjoy your wonderful smoothie!

Nutrition:

Calories 358 | Fat 19.8 g | Carbohydrates 1.3 g | Sugar 0.4 g | Protein 41.9 g | Cholesterol 131 mg

Citrus Detox Juice

Preparation Time: 10 minutes | Cooking Time: 0 minutes | Servings: 4

Ingredients:

- Water (3 C.)

- Lemon (1, Sliced)

- Grapefruit (1, Sliced)

- Orange (1, Sliced)

Directions:

- Begin by peeling and slicing up your fruit. Once this is done, place it in a pitcher of water and infuse the water overnight.

Nutrition:

Calories: 269 | Total Carbohydrate: 2 g | Cholesterol: 3 mg | Total Fat: 14 g | Fiber: 2 g | Protein: 7 g | Sodium: 183 mg

Metabolism Water

Preparation Time: 10 minutes | Cooking Time: 0 minutes | Servings: 1

Ingredients:

• Water (3 C.)

• Cucumber (1, Sliced)

• Lemon (1, Sliced)

• Mint (2 Leaves)

• Ice

Directions:

• All you will have to do is get out a pitcher, place all of the ingredients in, and allow the ingredients to soak overnight for maximum benefits!

Nutrition:

Calories: 301 | Total Carbohydrate: 2 g | Cholesterol: 13 mg | Total Fat: 17 g | Fiber: 4 g | Protein: 8 g | Sodium: 201 mg

Stress Relief Detox Drink

Preparation Time: 5 minutes | Cooking Time: 0 minutes | Servings: 1

Ingredients:

• Water (1 Pitcher)

• Mint

• Lemon (1, Sliced)

• Basil

• Strawberries (1 C., Sliced)

• Ice

Directions:

• When you are ready, take all of the ingredients and place them into a pitcher of water overnight and enjoy the next day.

Nutrition:

Calories: 189 | Total Carbohydrate: 2 g | Cholesterol: 73 mg | Total Fat: 17 g | Fiber: 0 g | Protein: 7 g | Sodium: 163 mg

Strawberry Pink Drink

Preparation Time: 10 minutes | Cooking Time: 5 minutes | Servings: 4

Ingredients:

• Water (1 C., Boiling)

• Sugar (2 T.)

• Acai Tea Bag (1)

• Coconut Milk (1 C.)

• Frozen Strawberries (1/2 C.)

Directions:

• You will begin by boiling your cup of water and steep the teabag in for at least five minutes.

• When the tea is set, add in the sugar and coconut milk. Be sure to stir well to spread the sweetness throughout the tea.

• Finally, add in your strawberries, and you can enjoy your freshly made pink drink!

Nutrition:

Calories: 321 | Total Carbohydrate: 2 g | Cholesterol: 13 mg | Total Fat: 17 g | Fiber: 2 g | Protein: 9 g | Sodium: 312 mg

Lavender and Mint Iced Tea

Preparation Time: 5 minutes | Cooking Time: 10 minutes | Servings: 8 servings

Ingredients:

• 8 cups of water

• 1/3 cup of dried lavender buds

• ¼ cup of mint

Directions:

• Add the mint and lavender to a pot and set this aside.

• Add eight cups of boiling water to the pot. Sweeten to taste, cover, and let steep for ten

minutes. Strain, chill and serve.

Tips:

• Use a sweetener of your choice when making this iced tea.

• Add spirits to turn this iced tea into a summer cocktail.

Nutrition:

Calories 266 | Carbs: 9.3g | Protein: 20.9g | Fat: 16.1g

Pear Lemonade

Preparation Time: 5 minutes | Cooking Time: 30 minutes | Servings: 2 servings

Ingredients:

- ½ cup of pear, peeled and diced

- 1 cup of freshly squeezed lemon juice

- ½ cup of chilled water

Directions:

• Add all the ingredients into a blender and pulse until it has all been combined. The pear does make the lemonade frothy, but this will settle.

• Place in the refrigerator to cool and then serve.

Tips:

• Keep stored in a sealed container in the refrigerator for up to four days.

• Pop the fresh lemon in the microwave for ten minutes before juicing, you can extract more juice if you do this.

Nutrition:

Calories: 160 | Carbs: 6.3g | Protein: 2.9g | Fat: 13.6g

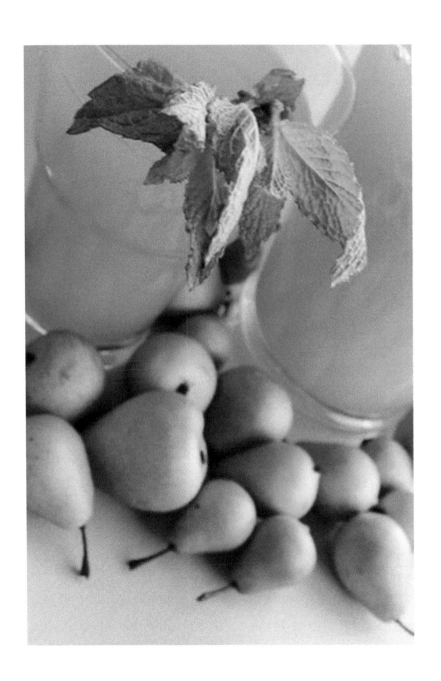

Energizing Ginger Detox Tonic

Preparation Time: 15 minutes | Cooking Time: 10 minutes | Servings:

Ingredients:

- 1/2 teaspoon of grated ginger, fresh

- 1 small lemon slice

- 1/8 teaspoon of cayenne pepper

- 1/8 teaspoon of ground turmeric

- 1/8 teaspoon of ground cinnamon

- 1 teaspoon of maple syrup

- 1 teaspoon of apple cider vinegar

- 2 cups of boiling water

Directions:

- Pour the boiling water into a small saucepan, add and stir the ginger, then let it rest for 8 to 10 minutes, before covering the pan.

• Pass the mixture through a strainer and into the liquid, add the cayenne pepper, turmeric, cinnamon and stir properly.

• Add the maple syrup, vinegar, and lemon slice.

• Add and stir an infused lemon and serve immediately.

Nutrition:

Calories 443 | Carbs:9.7 g | Protein: 62.8g | Fat: 16.9g

Strawberry Shake

Preparation Time: 10 minutes | Cooking Time: 10 minutes | Servings: 2

Ingredients:

• 1½ cups fresh strawberries, hulled

• 1 large frozen banana, peeled

• 2 scoops unsweetened vegan vanilla protein powder

• 2 tablespoons hemp seeds

• 2 cups unsweetened hemp milk

Directions:

• In a high-speed blender, place all the ingredients and pulse until creamy.

• Pour into two glasses and serve immediately.

Nutrition:

Calories: 259 | Fat: 3g | Protein: 10g | Sugar: 2g

Chocolatey Banana Shake

Preparation Time: 10 minutes | Cooking Time: 10 minutes | Servings: 2

Ingredients:

- 2 medium frozen bananas, peeled

- 4 dates, pitted

- 4 tablespoons peanut butter

- 4 tablespoons rolled oats

- 2 tablespoons cacao powder

- 2 tablespoons chia seeds

- 2 cups unsweetened soymilk

Directions:

- Place all the ingredients in a high-speed blender and pulse until creamy.

- Pour into two glasses and serve immediately.

Nutrition:

Calories: 502 | Fat: 4g | Protein: 11g | Sugar: 9g

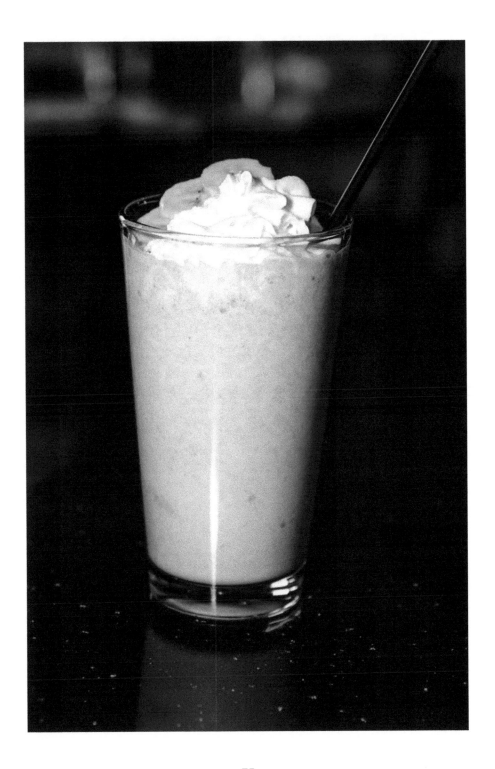

Fruity Tofu Smoothie

Preparation Time: 10 minutes | Cooking Time: 10 minutes | Servings: 2

Ingredients:

- 12 ounces silken tofu, pressed and drained

- 2 medium bananas, peeled

- 1½ cups fresh blueberries

- 1 tablespoon maple syrup

- 1½ cups unsweetened soymilk

- ¼ cup of ice cubes

Directions:

- Place all the ingredients in a high-speed blender and pulse until creamy.

- Pour into two glasses and serve immediately.

Nutrition:

Calories 235 | Carbohydrates: 1.9g | Protein: 14.3g | Fat: 18.9g

Green Fruity Smoothie

Preparation Time: 10 minutes | Cooking Time: 10 minutes | Servings: 2

Ingredients:

• 1 cup of frozen mango, peeled, pitted, and chopped

• 1 large frozen banana, peeled

• 2 cups fresh baby spinach

• 1 scoop unsweetened vegan vanilla protein powder

• ¼ cup pumpkin seeds

• 2 tablespoons hemp hearts

• 1½ cups unsweetened almond milk

Directions:

• In a high-speed blender, place all the ingredients and pulse until creamy.

• Pour into two glasses and serve immediately.

Nutrition:

Calories 206 | Carbohydrates: 1.3g | Protein: 23.5g | Fat: 11.9g

Protein Latte

Preparation Time: 10 minutes | Cooking Time: 10 minutes | Servings: 2

Ingredients:

• 2 cups hot brewed coffee

• 1¼ cups coconut milk

• 2 teaspoons coconut oil

• 2 scoops unsweetened vegan vanilla protein powder

Directions:

• Place all the ingredients in a high-speed blender and pulse until creamy.

• Pour into two serving mugs and serve immediately.

Nutrition:

Calories 483 | Carbs: 5.2g | Protein: 45.2g | Fat: 31.2g

Health Boosting Juices

Preparation Time: 10 minutes | Cooking Time: 15 minutes | Servings: 2

Ingredients for a red juice:

• 4 beetroots, quartered

• 2 cups of strawberries

• 2 cups of blueberries

• Ingredients for an orange juice:

• 4 green or red apples, halved

• 10 carrots

• ½ lemon, peeled

• 1∥ of ginger

• Ingredients for a yellow juice:

• 2 green or red apples, quartered

• 4 oranges, peeled and halved

• ½ lemon, peeled

• 1∥ of ginger

Ingredients for lime juice:

- 6 stalks of celery

- 1 cucumber

- 2 green apples, quartered

- 2 pears, quartered

Ingredients for a green juice:

- ½ a pineapple, peeled and sliced

- 8 leaves of kale

- 2 fresh bananas, peeled

Directions:

- Juice all ingredients in a juicer, chill, and serve.

Nutrition:

Calories 316 | Carbs: 13.5g | Protein: 37.8g | Fat: 12.2g

Thai Iced Tea

Preparation Time: 5 minutes | Cooking Time: 10 minutes | Servings: 4

Ingredients:

- 4 cups of water

- 1 can of light coconut milk (14 oz.)

- ¼ cup of maple syrup

- ¼ cup of muscovado sugar

- 1 teaspoon of vanilla extract

- 2 tablespoons of loose-leaf black tea

Directions:

- In a large saucepan, over medium heat bring the water to a boil.

- Turn off the heat and add in the tea, cover and let steep for five minutes.

- Strain the tea into a bowl or jug. Add the maple syrup, muscovado sugar, and vanilla extract.

Give it a good whisk to blend all the ingredients.

• Set in the refrigerator to chill. Upon serving, pour ¾ of the tea into each glass, top with coconut milk, and stir.

Tips:

• Add a shot of dark rum to turn this iced tea into a cocktail.

• You could substitute the coconut milk for almond or rice milk too.

Nutrition:

Calories 844 | Carbohydrates: 2.3g | Protein: 21.6g | Fat: 83.1g

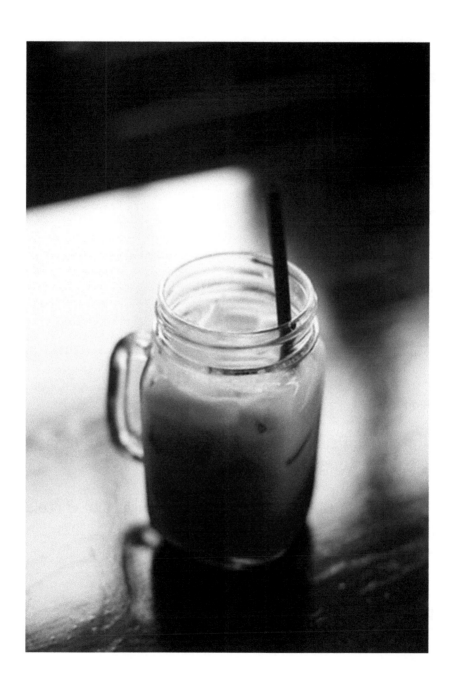

Hot Chocolate

Preparation Time: 5 minutes | Cooking Time: 15 minutes | Servings: 2

Ingredients:

• Pinch of brown sugar

• 2 cups of milk, soy or almond, unsweetened

• 2 tablespoons of cocoa powder

• ½ cup of vegan chocolate

Directions:

• In a medium saucepan, over medium heat gently bring the milk to a boil. Whisk in the cocoa powder.

• Remove from the heat, add a pinch of sugar and chocolate. Give it a good stir until smooth, serve, and enjoy.

Tips:

• You may substitute the almond or soy milk for coconut milk too.

Nutrition:

Calories 452 | Carbs: 29.8g | Protein: 15.2g | Fat: 30.2g

Chai and Chocolate Milkshake

Preparation Time: 5 minutes | Cooking Time: 15 minutes | Servings: 2 servings

Ingredients:

• 1 and ½ cups of almond milk, sweetened or unsweetened

• 3 bananas, peeled and frozen 12 hours before use

• 4 dates, pitted

• 1 and ½ teaspoons of chocolate powder, sweetened or unsweetened

• ½ teaspoon of vanilla extract

• ½ teaspoon of cinnamon

• ¼ teaspoon of ground ginger

• Pinch of ground cardamom

• Pinch of ground cloves

• Pinch of ground nutmeg

• ½ cup of ice cubes

Directions:

• Add all the ingredients to a blender except for the ice-cubes. Pulse until smooth and creamy, add the ice-cubes, pulse a few more times and serve.

Tips:

• The dates provide enough sweetness to the recipe, however, you are welcome to add maple syrup or honey for a sweeter drink.

Nutrition:

Calories 452 | Carbs: 29.8g | Protein: 15.2g | Fat: 30.2g

Lemon Infused Water

Preparation Time: 10 minutes | Cooking Time: 2 hours | Servings: 12

Ingredients:

• 2 cups of coconut sugar

• 2 cups of lemon juice

• 3 quarts of water

Directions:

• Pour water into a 6-quarts slow cooker and stir the sugar and lemon juice properly.

• Then plug in the slow cooker and let it cook on a high heat setting for 2 hours or until it is heated thoroughly.

• Serve the drink hot or cold.

Nutrition:

Calories 523 | Carbohydrates: 4.6g | Protein: 47.9g | Fat: 34.8g

Soothing Ginger Tea Drink

Preparation Time: 5 minutes | Cooking Time: 2 hours 20 minutes | Servings: 8

Ingredients:

• 1 tablespoon of minced ginger root

• 2 tablespoons of honey

• 15 green tea bags

• 32 fluid ounce of white grape juice

• 2 quarts of boiling water

Directions:

• Pour water into a 4-quarts slow cooker, immerse tea bags, cover the cooker, and let stand for 10 minutes.

• After 10 minutes, remove and discard tea bags and stir in the remaining ingredients.

• Return cover to the slow cooker, let cook at high heat setting for 2 hours or until heated through.

• When done, strain the liquid and serve hot or cold.

Nutrition:

Calories 232 | Carbs: 7.9g | Protein: 15.9g | Fat: 15.1g

Ginger Cherry Cider

Preparation Time: 1 hour 5 minutes | Cooking Time: 3 hours | Servings: 16

Ingredients:

• 2 knobs of ginger, each about 2 inches

• 6-ounce of cherry gelatin

• 4 quarts of apple cider

Directions:

• Using a 6-quarts slow cooker, pour the apple cider and add the ginger.

• Stir, then cover the slow cooker with its lid. let it cook for 3 hours at the high heat setting or until it is heated thoroughly.

• Then add and stir the gelatin properly, then continue cooking for another hour.

• When done, remove the ginger and serve the drink hot or cold.

Nutrition:

Calories 78 | Carbs: 13.2g | Protein: 2.8g | Fat: 1.5g

Colorful Infused Water

Preparation Time: 5 minutes | Cooking Time: 1 hour | Servings: 8 servings

Ingredients:

- 1 cup of strawberries, fresh or frozen

- 1 cup of blueberries, fresh or frozen

- 1 tablespoon of baobab powder

- 1 cup of ice cubes

- 4 cups of sparkling water

Directions:

- In a large water jug, add in the sparkling water, ice cubes, and baobab powder. Give it a good stir.

- Add in the strawberries and blueberries and cover the infused water, store in the refrigerator for one hour before serving.

Tips:

- Store for 12 hours for optimum taste and nutritional benefits.

• Instead of using strawberries and blueberries, add slices of lemon and six mint leaves, one cup of mangoes or cherries, or half a cup of leafy greens such as kale and/or spinach.

Nutrition:

Calories 163 | Carbs: 4.1g | Protein: 1.7g | Fat: 15.5g

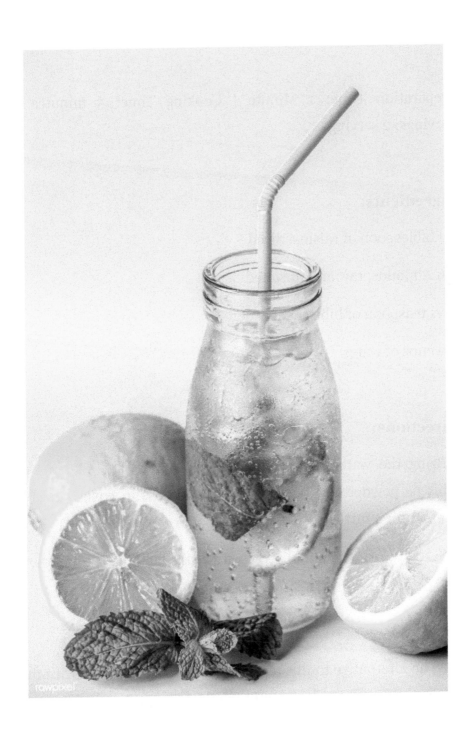

Hibiscus Tea

Preparation Time: 1 Minute | Cooking Time: 5 minutes | Servings: 2 servings

Ingredients:

• 1 tablespoon of raisins, diced

• 6 Almonds, raw and unsalted

• ½ teaspoon of hibiscus powder

• 2 cups of water

Directions:

• Bring the water to a boil in a small saucepan, add in the hibiscus powder and raisins. Give it a good stir, cover, and let simmer for a further two minutes.

• Strain into a teapot and serve with a side helping of almonds.

Tips:

• As an alternative to this tea, do not strain it and serve with the raisin pieces still swirling around in the teacup.

• You could also serve this tea chilled for those hotter days.

• Double or triple the recipe to provide you with iced-tea to enjoy during the week without having to make a fresh pot each time.

Nutrition:

Calories 139 | Carbohydrates: 2.7g | Protein: 8.7g | Fat: 10.3

Lemon and Rosemary Iced Tea

Preparation Time: 5 minutes | Cooking Time: 10 minutes | Servings: 4 servings

Ingredients:

• 4 cups of water

• 4 earl grey tea bags

• ¼ cup of sugar

• 2 lemons

• 1 sprig of rosemary

Directions:

• Peel the two lemons and set the fruit aside.

• In a medium saucepan, over medium heat combine the water, sugar, and lemon peels. Bring this to a boil.

• Remove from the heat and place the rosemary and tea into the mixture. Cover the saucepan and steep for five minutes.

• Add the juice of the two peeled lemons to the mixture, strain, chill, and serve.

• Tips:

• Skip the sugar and use honey to taste.

• Do not squeeze the tea bags as they can cause the tea to become bitter.

Nutrition:

Calories 229 | Carbs: 33.2g | Protein: 31.1g | Fat: 10.2g

Fragrant Spiced Coffee

Preparation Time: 10 minutes | Cooking Time: 3 hours | Servings: 8

Ingredients:

- 4 cinnamon sticks, each about 3 inches long

- 1 1/2 teaspoons of whole cloves

- 1/3 cup of honey

- 2-ounce of chocolate syrup

- 1/2 teaspoon of anise extract

- 8 cups of brewed coffee

Directions:

- Pour the coffee into a 4-quarts slow cooker and pour in the remaining ingredients except for cinnamon and stir properly.

- Wrap the whole cloves in cheesecloth and tie its corners with strings.

- Immerse this cheesecloth bag in the liquid present in the slow cooker and cover it with the lid.

- Then plug in the slow cooker and let it cook on the low heat setting for 3 hours or until heated thoroughly.

- When done, discard the cheesecloth bag and serve.

Nutrition:

Calories 136 | Fat 12.6 g | Carbohydrates 4.1 g | Sugar 0.5 g | Protein 10.3 g | Cholesterol 88 mg

Bracing Coffee Smoothie

Preparation Time: 5 minutes | Cooking Time: 5 minutes | Servings: 1

Ingredients:

• 1 banana, sliced and frozen

• ½ cup strong brewed coffee

• ½ cup milk

• ¼ cup rolled oats

• 1 tsp nut butter

Directions:

• Mix all the ingredients until smooth.

• Enjoy your morning drink!

Nutrition:

Calories 414 | Fat 20.6 g | Carbohydrates 5.6 g | Sugar 1.3 g | Protein 48.8 g | Cholesterol 58 mg

Ginger Smoothie with Citrus and Mint

Preparation Time: 5 minutes | Cooking Time: 3 minutes | Servings: 3

Ingredients:

- 1 head Romaine lettuce, chopped into 4 chunks

- 2 Tbsp hemp seeds

- 5 mandarin oranges, peeled

- 1 banana, frozen

- 1 carrot

- 2-3 mint leaves

- ½ piece of ginger root, peeled

- 1 cup of water

- ¼ lemon, peeled

- ½ cup ice

Directions:

• Put all the smoothie ingredients in a blender and blend until smooth.

• Enjoy!

Nutrition:

Calories 101 | Fat 4 g | Carbohydrates 14 g | Sugar 1 g | Protein 2 g | Cholesterol 3 mg

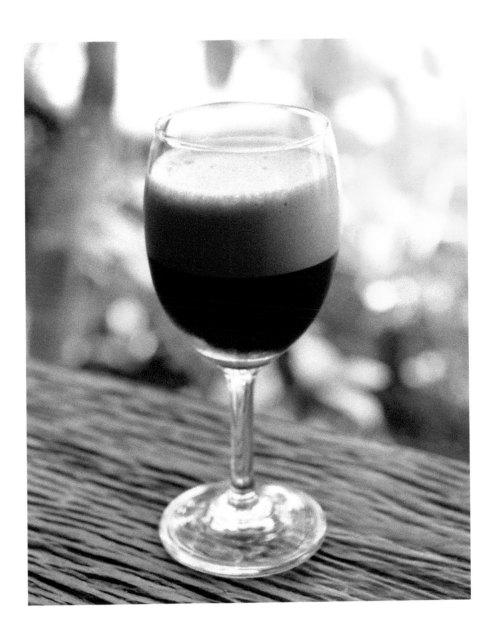

Lightning Source UK Ltd.
Milton Keynes UK
UKHW020654100621
385265UK00005B/150